Salads and Brunch

GW01246705

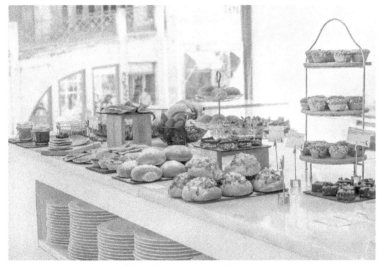

Cookbook Vol.2

This book contains low-fat, quick and easy recipes for beginners, ideated to boost your lifestyle from the awakening and balance your daily supply. Taste the whole Mediterranean diet in some fast and mouth-watering fresh recipes!

Kumar Ortega

Table of Contents

Welcome, dear reader!

This is my purpose to you.

This cookbook is a creation born from a researcher of the wellness. It's finalized to increase your energies and to let you live a happier life, without the heaviness of the modern kitchen.

In this book, you'll find my knowledge on how to keep your body and mind faculties active, productive and efficient.

Jump into a world of good habits and natural foods, if you want to discover the real deepness of your overall wellness.

Nevertheless, you'll learn new ideas, discover tastes of all around the world and change your meal plan in better.

Each of these dishes is thought to:

1 - Let you wake up full of energies and keep this boost for all day long

Thanks to light and natural greens as dinner and a high nutrient supply as brunch, you'll sleep better and be full of energies during the day.

2 - Lose the excessive weight and keep your moral up

As soon as you start to eat better and do physical activity, the leftover fat will disappear from your body and your image will finally become as you wish!

3 - Improve your skills and surprise your friends

Learn some new recipes taken from the worldwide tradition and twisted by a proper chef, only to let you discover modern tastes.

Salad Recipes

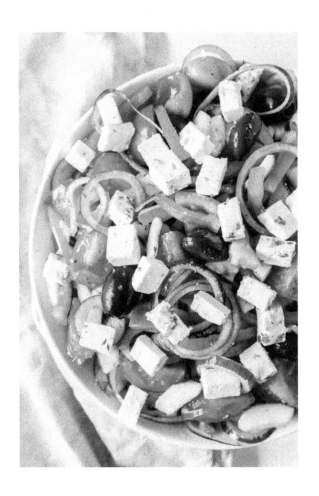

Spinaches and Strawberries Salad

Serves 8 pax

Ingredients

- 1/4 cup white wine vinegar
- 2 bunches spinach, rinsed
- 2 tablespoons sesame seeds
- 1 tablespoon poppy seeds
- 4 cups sliced strawberries
- 1/2 cup vegetable oil
- 1/2 cup white sugar
- 1/4 teaspoon paprika

Procedure

1. Mix strawberries and spinach in a big bowl.
2. Combine poppy seeds, sesame seeds, paprika, sugar, vinegar, and oil in a medium-sized bowl.
3. Pour over the strawberries and spinach, mix to coat.
4. Serve.

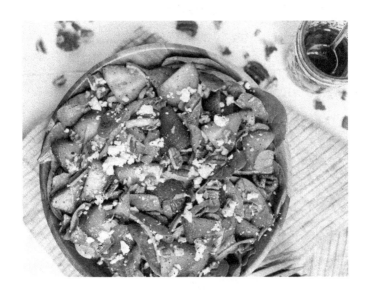

Spring Salad

Serves 6 pax

Ingredients

- 1 head romaine lettuce, torn
- 1 cup alfalfa sprouts
- 1 red bell pepper, chopped
- 2 teaspoons vegetable oil
- 1 cup raspberry vinaigrette salad dressing
- 1/2 bunch fresh spinach, chopped
- 3 roma tomatoes, chopped
- 8 ounces fresh mushrooms, sliced

Procedure

1. Set up the oven broiler to preheat.
2. Apply oil to the pepper with a brush and put it on a baking sheet. Broil until black splotches turn up on all sides while sometimes flipping.
3. Take away from the heat and use plastic to wrap it tightly. Set aside about 15 minutes then get rid of the pulp and seeds, and chop.
4. Toss raspberry vinaigrette, sprouts, mushrooms, tomatoes, spinach, romaine lettuce and roasted red pepper together in a big bowl.
5. Serve.

Carrot Ambrosia Salad

Serves 8 pax

Ingredients

- 1/2 cup raisins
- 1/2 cup coconut
- 1/2 cup yogurt
- 1/2 cup pineapple tidbits in pineapple juice, undrained
- 2 tablespoons honey, or to taste
- 4 cups spiral-sliced carrots

Procedure

1. In a bowl, stir together honey, coconut, raisins, pineapple and yogurt, then put in carrots.
2. Stir until ingredients are blended completely.
3. Chill for a half hour until cold, then stir again before serving.

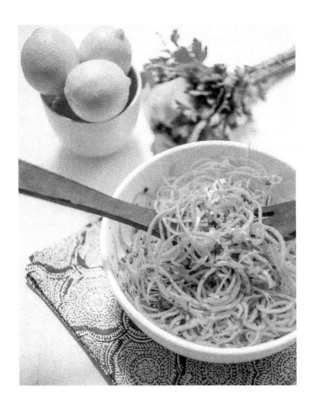

Mushroom and spinaches Salad

Serves 4 pax

Ingredients

- 2 teaspoons white sugar
- 4 slices bacon
- 2 eggs
- 1 pound spinach
- 1/4 pound fresh mushrooms, sliced
- 2 tablespoons cider vinegar
- 2 tablespoons water
- 1/2 teaspoon salt

Procedure

1. Put bacon in a big, deep skillet. Cook over moderately high heat until equally browned. Crumble and set aside, save 2 tbsp. bacon fat.
2. In a saucepan, add eggs, and pour in cold water to cover totally. Bring water to a boil. Cover, take away from heat, and allow eggs to stand in hot water for about 10 to 12 minutes.
3. Take the eggs out of hot water, cool, peel and slice into wedges.
4. Bring 2 tbsp. bacon fat back to the skillet, then stir in salt, water, vinegar and sugar, keep it warm.
5. Rinse and remove stems from spinach, dry completely and crumble into pieces in a salad bowl.
6. Drizzle the warm dressing over and toss well to coat.
7. Place bacon and mushrooms on top of the salad, decorate with egg.

Tabbouleh

Serves 6 pax

Ingredients

- 1/2 cup bulgur
- 1/8 teaspoon cayenne pepper
- 2 lemon juice
- 1/2 cup mint
- 6 tablespoons extra-virgin olive oil
- Salt and pepper
- 1 cup parsley
- 2 scallions
- 3 tomatoes

Procedure

1. Toss tomatoes with 1/4 teaspoon salt using a fine-mesh strainer set over bowl and let drain, tossing occasionally, for 30 minutes. Reserve 2 tablespoons drained tomato juice.

2. Toss bulgur with 2 tablespoons lemon juice and reserved tomato juice in a container and allow to sit until grains start to become tender, 30 to 40 minutes.

3. Beat remaining 2 tablespoons lemon juice, oil, cayenne, and 1/4 teaspoon salt together in a big container.

4. Put in tomatoes, bulgur, parsley, mint, and scallions and toss gently to combine. Cover and allow to sit at room temperature until flavors have blended and bulgur is tender, about 1 hour.

5. Before serving, toss salad to recombine and sprinkle with salt and pepper to taste.

6. Serve.

Tuna Olive Salad

Serves 6 pax

Ingredients

- 1 garlic clove
- 1 tablespoon parsley
- 1/2 cup pimento-stuffed green olives
- 5 tablespoons extra-virgin olive oil
- Salt and pepper to taste to taste
- 15 ounces cannellini beans, rinsed
- 12 ounces cherry tomatoes
- 12 ounces tuna steaks
- 4 tablespoons lemon juice
- 5 cups arugula

Procedure

1. Beat olives, lemon juice, parsley, and garlic together in a big container. Whisking continuously, slowly drizzle in 5 tablespoons oil. Sprinkle with Salt and pepper to taste to taste.

2. Pat tuna dry using paper towels and sprinkle with Salt and pepper to taste. Heat residual 1 tablespoon oil in 12-inch non-stick frying pan on moderate to high heat until just smoking.

3. Cook tuna until thoroughly browned and translucent red at center when checked with tip of paring knife and registers 110 degrees (for rare), approximately two minutes each side.

4. Move to slicing board and slice into 1/2inch-thick slices. Beat dressing to re-emulsify, then drizzle 1 tablespoon dressing over tuna.

5. Put in arugula, tomatoes, and beans to a container with remaining dressing and gently toss to combine.

6. Sprinkle with Salt and pepper to taste to taste. Divide salad among plates and top with tuna. Serve.

Green Salad

Serves 4 pax

Ingredients

- 1/2 garlic clove
- 8 ounces lettuce
- 2 tbsp Extra-virgin olive oil
- Salt and pepper to taste to taste
- 1 tbsp Vinegar

Procedure

1. Take a salad bowl and coat its inside with garlic. Put in lettuce. Cautiously sprinkle lettuce with a little oil.

2. Slowly toss the contents of the bowl. Carry on drizzling with oil and toss gently until greens are mildly coated and barely starting to shine.

3. Drizzle with small amounts of vinegar, salt, and pepper to taste and toss gently to coat.

4. Serve.

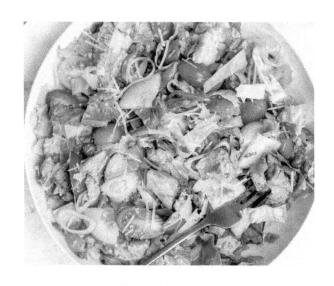

Kale Sweet Potato Salad

Serves 8 pax

Ingredients

- 1 pound sweet potatoes
- 12 ounces Tuscan kale
- 1/3 cup pecans
- 1/2 head radicchio
- Salt and pepper to taste
- Shaved Parmesan cheese
- 2 teaspoons extra-virgin olive oil
- 4 tbsp vinaigrette

Procedure

1. Place the oven rack in the center of the oven and pre-heat your oven to 400 degrees. Toss sweet potatoes with oil and sprinkle with Salt and pepper to taste.

2. Arrange potatoes in one layer in rimmed baking sheet and roast until browned, 25 to 30 minutes, flipping potatoes halfway through roasting. Move to plate and allow to cool for 20 minutes.

3. In the meantime, heavily squeeze and massage kale with hands until leaves are uniformly darkened and slightly wilted, about 1 minute.

4. Put in potatoes, kale, and radicchio to vinaigrette and gently toss to coat.

5. Sprinkle with Salt and pepper to taste to taste. Move to serving platter and drizzle with pecans and shaved Parmesan to taste.

Spinach Feta Pistachio Salad

Serves6 Servings

Ingredients

- 1 ounce feta cheese
- 2 teaspoons sugar
- 1 strip lemon zest plus 2 tablespoons juice
- 1 shallot
- 6 radishes
- Salt and pepper to taste
- 10 ounces curly-leaf spinach
- 3 tablespoons pistachios
- 3 tablespoons extra-virgin olive oil

Procedure

1. Place feta on plate and freeze until mildly stiff, about fifteen minutes.
2. Cook oil, lemon zest, shallot, and sugar in Dutch oven over moderate to low heat until shallot is softened, approximately five minutes.
3. Remove from the heat, discard zest and mix in lemon juice. Put in spinach, cover, and let steam off heat until it just begins to wilt, approximately half a minute. Move spinach mixture and liquid left in pot to big container.
4. Put in radishes, pistachios, and chilled feta and toss to combine.
5. Sprinkle with Salt and pepper to taste to taste.
6. Serve.

Tangy Salad

Serves 6 pax

Ingredients

- 1 small shallot, minced
- 1 teaspoon Dijon mustard
- 1/2 cup smoked almonds, chopped coarse
- 2/3 cup chopped pitted dates
- 1 small head radicchio, cored and sliced thin
- 5 tablespoons extra-virgin olive oil
- Salt and pepper to taste
- 1 Teaspoon sugar
- 2 red grapefruits
- 3 oranges

Procedure

1. Cut away peel and pith from grapefruits and oranges.
2. Cut each fruit in half from pole to pole, then slice crosswise 1/4 inch thick.
3. Move to a container, toss with sugar and 1/2 teaspoon salt, and allow to sit for about fifteen minutes.
4. Drain fruit in fine-mesh strainer set over bowl, reserving 2 tablespoons juice. Arrange fruit on serving platter and drizzle with oil.
5. Beat reserved juice, shallot, and mustard together in medium bowl. Put in radicchio, 1/3 cup dates, and 1/4 cup almonds and gently toss to coat. Sprinkle with Salt and pepper to taste to taste.
6. Arrange radicchio mixture over fruit, leaving 1-inch border of fruit around edges.
7. Sprinkle with remaining 1/3 cup dates and remaining 1/4 cup almonds. Serve.

Tri-Balsamic Salad

Ingredients

- 1 tablespoon balsamic vinegar
- 1 head Belgian endive, cut into 2-inch pieces
- 1 small head radicchio, cored and cut
- 3 tablespoons extra-virgin olive oil
- Salt and pepper to taste
- 1 teaspoon red wine vinegar
- 3 ounces baby arugula

Procedure

1. Gently toss radicchio, endive, and arugula together in a big container.
2. Beat balsamic vinegar, red wine vinegar, 1/8 teaspoon salt, and pinch pepper together in a small-sized container.
3. Whisking continuously, slowly drizzle in oil.
4. Drizzle vinaigrette over salad and gently toss to coat.
5. Drizzle with Salt and pepper to taste to taste. Serve.

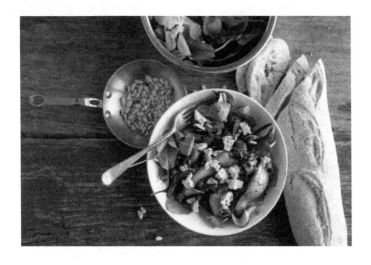

Algerian Salad

Serves 6 pax

Ingredients

- 1/2 cup pitted oil-cured black olives, quartered
- 4 blood oranges Salt and pepper to taste
- 1/4 cup coarsely chopped fresh mint
- 1/4 cup extra-virgin olive oil
- 2 fennel bulbs, stalks discarded, bulbs halved, cored, and sliced thin
- 2 tablespoons lemon juice

Procedure

1. Cut away peel and pith from oranges. Quarter oranges, then slice crosswise into 1/4-inch-thick pieces.
2. Mix oranges, fennel, olives, and mint in a big container.
3. Beat lemon juice, 1/4 teaspoon salt, and 1/8 teaspoon pepper together in a small sized container.
4. Whisking continuously, slowly drizzle in oil.
5. Sprinkle dressing over salad and gently toss to coat. Sprinkle with Salt and pepper to taste to taste.
6. Serve.

Asparagus Salad

Serves 6 pax

Ingredients

For the pesto

- 1/2 cup extra-virgin olive oil
- 1/4 cup basil leaves
- 1/4 cup grated sheep cheese
- 1 garlic clove
- 1 teaspoon grated lemon zest plus 2 teaspoons juice

For the salad

- 3/4 cup hazelnuts, toasted, skinned, and chopped
- 2 oranges
- 2 pounds asparagus, trimmed
- 4 ounces feta cheese, crumbled

Procedure

For the Pesto

1. Process basil, Pecorino, lemon zest and juice, garlic, and 3/4 teaspoon salt using a food processor until finely chopped, approximately half a minute, scraping down sides of the container as required. Move to big container.
2. Mix in oil and sprinkle with Salt and pepper to taste to taste.

For the Salad

3. Chop asparagus tips from stalks into 3/4-inch-long pieces. Cut asparagus stalks 1/8 inch thick on bias into approximate 2-inch lengths. Cut away the peel and pith from oranges.
4. Holding fruit over bowl, use paring knife to cut between membranes to release segments.
5. Put in asparagus tips and stalks, orange segments, feta, and hazelnuts to pesto and toss to combine.
6. Sprinkle with Salt and pepper to taste to taste.
7. Serve.

Healty Brunch

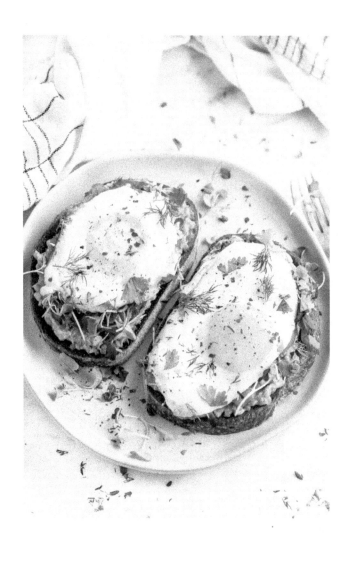

Peach Smoothie

Serves 1 pax

Ingredients

- 0.5 cups Milk
- 0.5 cups Crushed ice
- 1 Tbsp Orange juice
- Stevia or artificial sweetener of your choice
- 1 Peach

Procedure

1. Peel and remove the pit from the peaches if you are using fresh ones.
2. Slice them into wedges for easy blending.
3. Place each of the fixings in a blender.
4. Mix until it's creamy.
5. Serve promptly for freshness.

Blueberry Almond Smoothie

Serves 3 pax

Ingredients

- Half Lime juice
- 2 Tbsp Tightly packed fresh mint leaves
- 1.5 cups Almond milk
- 1 cup Ice
- 1 Tbsp Raw honey
- 1.5 cups blueberries
- 1 Tbsp Ground flaxseeds
- 2 Tbsp Almond flour

Procedure

1. Puree each of the fixings in a blender until they are creamy smooth.
2. Pour one cup in each of the three glasses and serve immediately.

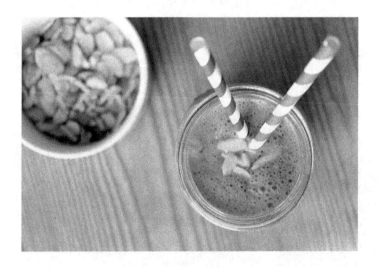

Puff Pastry Toast

Serves 8 pax

Ingredients

- 3 cups unbleached all-purpose flour
- cup plain bleached cake flour
- 6 sticks unsalted butter, chilled
- 2 teaspoons salt 1 cup ice water

Procedure

1. Dice butter sticks into 1/2 -inch cubes. Put flour in mixing bowl. Add butter and salt. Blend flour and butter together until butter broken into small lumps.

2. Blend in water and mix until dough clumps roughly together but butter pieces remain the same. On a lightly floured work surface, quickly push, pat and roll dough to form a 12-inch by 18-inch rectangle. Lightly flour top of dough.

3. Using a pastry sheet, flip the bottom of the rectangle up over the middle. Flip the top of the rectangle down to cover it. Lift the dough away from the work surface using a pastry sheet.

4. Return the dough to the work surface. Set it with the top flap to your right. Lightly flour top of the dough, and push, pat and roll again into a rectangle.

5. Repeat folding as above. (Each "roll-and-fold" operation is called a "turn". Repeat process 2 more times. (4 "turns" in total). After the last "turn" you will see flakes of butter scattered below the surface on the dough. Wrap dough in plastic wrap and place in a plastic bag. Refrigerate 40 minutes.

6. Repeat "turn" process 2 more times. Let dough rest 30 minutes. Dough is ready for baking when rubbery and difficult to roll.

7. Pre-heat oven to 400°F. Unfold pastry on a lightly floured work surface. Cut pastry sheet into 5-inch squares. Place pastry squares on a baking sheet. Prick the pastry squares with a fork. Bake for 20 minutes or until the toasted pastry squares are toasted golden brown.

8. Let it cool and serve.

Spinaches and Cereals Salad

Serves 8 pax

Ingredients

- 1/2 pound crumbled feta cheese
- 1 (16 ounce) package uncooked orzo pasta
- 1 (10 ounce) package baby spinach leaves, finely chopped
- 1/2 cup olive oil
- 1/2 cup balsamic vinegar
- 1/2 red onion, finely chopped
- 3/4 cup pine nuts
- 1/2 teaspoon dried basil
- 1/4 teaspoon ground white pepper

Procedure

8. Boil a big pot of lightly salted water; put in orzo. Cook for 8-10 mins until it is al dente; drain.

9. Rinse orzo using cold water. Move to a big bowl.

10. Mix in white pepper, spinach, basil, feta, pine nuts, and onion.

11. Drizzle with balsamic vinegar and onion; toss to coat.

12. Let it chill in the refrigerator then serve.

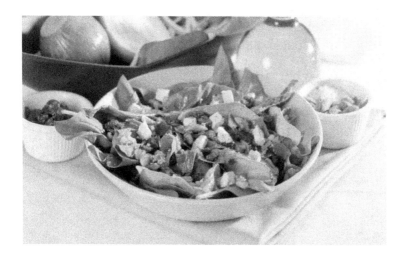

Breakfast Pizza

Serves 2 pax

Ingredients

- 1 Tomato
- 0.25 cups Monterey Jack cheese
- 2 Whole-wheat English muffins
- 1 Tbsp Skim milk
- 0.5 cups Egg
- Half Red bell pepper
- 1 Button mushrooms
- 1 Green onion
- 1 tsp margarine

Procedure

1. Melt the margarine in a skillet using a med-high temperature setting, making sure it coats the bottom.
2. Stirring frequently, sauté the mushrooms, onions, and bell pepper until tender (3 min.).
3. Combine the egg substitute and milk in a small mixing container, then pour the mixture over the vegetables, lowering the heat to medium.
4. Cook, but don't stir, until it begins to set around the edge, then scrape the mixture to the center of the skillet, tilting the uncooked egg to the edge. Stir for 3 to 4 minutes, until it is all fully cooked.
5. Arrange the English muffin halves on a baking tray with the cut side up.
6. Top each with 1 Tbsp. cheese, then the egg mixture, then the remaining cheese. Place the tomato on top of the cheese.
7. Bake at 375°F until the cheese is melted, about 5 to 8 minutes.
8. Serve.

Lemon Blueberry Yogurt Parfait

Serves 4 pax

Ingredients

- 0.25 cups Almonds
- 1 cup Blueberries
- 2 Tbsp Vanilla extract
- 1 Lemon zest and juice
- 32 oz Greek yogurt

Procedure

1. Stir together the yogurt, lemon juice, lemon zest, Splenda, and vanilla.
2. Place 0.5 cups of the yogurt mixture in each of 4 serving dishes.
3. Place 0.25 cups of blueberries on top of each yogurt portion, then top the blueberries with another 0.5 cups yogurt mixture.
4. Top each serving with 1 Tbsp. of almonds.
5. Serve.

Green Artichoke Olive Salad

Ingredients

- 1 cup whole baby artichoke
- 1 ounce Asiago cheese
- 1/3 cup parsley leaves
- 1/3 cup pitted kalamata olives
- 1 romaine lettuce heart
- 5 tablespoons extra-virgin olive oil
- Salt and pepper to taste to taste
- 1 small garlic clove
- 4 tablespoons white wine vinegar
- 3 cups arugula

Procedure

1. Gently toss romaine, arugula, artichoke hearts, parsley, and olives together in a big container.
2. Beat vinegar, garlic, 1/4 teaspoon salt, and pinch pepper together in a small-sized container.
3. Whisking continuously, slowly drizzle in oil.
4. Sprinkle vinaigrette over salad and gently toss to coat.
5. Sprinkle with Salt and pepper to taste to taste.
6. Serve, topping individual portions with Asiago.

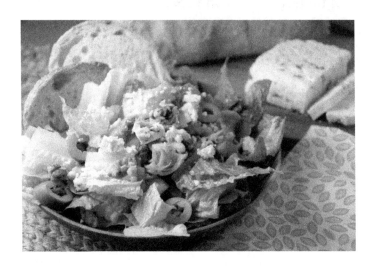

Parma Raw Ham with Fruits

Ingredients

- 1 tablespoon brown sugar
- 1 cup mixed tropical fruits like melon, papaya, pineapple, kiwis
- 4 tablespoons ricotta cheese
- 8 slices Parma raw ham
- 4 tablespoons wild honey
- 16 fresh figs

Procedure

1. Score the figs on top and gently squeeze to open them up into florets. Wrap prosciutto around the open figs.
2. Spoon ricotta into the openings. Sprinkle sugar on the ricotta, and place under hot grill.
3. Remove from heat when figs are warm and cheese begins to turn brown.
4. Drizzle honey over figs. Arrange with fresh tropical fruit slices.
5. Serve immediately.

Parma Raw Ham

Makes 1 whole Parma raw ham

Ingredients

- 12 ounces coarse sea salt warm water ·
- 1 pork leg with bone
- 1 horse-bone needle
- 1 meat hook
- 2 ounces grounded black pepper
- 10 ounces lard
- A cooking rope

Procedure

1. Trim away the fat and muscle from the ham until it is a traditional ham shape. Apply dry salt to exposed flesh and moistened salt to remaining skin.

2. Screw meat hook into the ceiling of a refrigerated chamber or walk-in refrigerator. Tie rope around middle of meat and hang the ham from the meat hook. Refrigerate at 39 degrees F for 1 week.

3. Brush away excess salt. Reapply salt and rehang the ham for 18 days. Lower temperature to 34 degrees F. Hang for 70 more days to "rest" the ham.

4. Wash the ham thoroughly with warm water and then air dry. Cure the ham for 3 months in an open, well aired room on a wooden rack.

5. Mix lard with a little salt and pepper to taste. Coat the ham with the lard to prevent it drying too quickly. Cure on the rack for another 6 months.

6. Insert horse-bone needle and check the smell and appearance of the ham. If it has a spicy, sweet aroma it is done.

7. Finish curing in cellar for 2 years and eat it.

Deviled Eggs

Serves 12 pax

Ingredients

- 1 pinch Salt
- 1 pinch Dry mustard
- 3 Scallions
- 1 tsp Freshly cracked black pepper
- 6 Tbsp mayonnaise
- 6 Eggs

Procedure

1. Gently arrange the eggs in a saucepan small enough that they are fairly tight together, so they don't bounce around and crack during the cooking process.

2. Cover the eggs with water and wait for them to boil. Immediately cover and transfer the pan from the burner.

3. Let them sit for 15 to 18 minutes, then drain and cover the eggs in cold water.

4. Peel the eggs, then vertically slice them in half.

5. Toss the egg yolks into a mixing container, then mix in the mustard, mayonnaise, pepper, and salt. Mash with a fork, mixing well.

6. Scoop the yolk mixture into the egg whites using a spoon.

7. Garnish them with scallions, if desired, and chill for about one hour.

8. Serve.

Gingerbread Oats

Serves 1 pax

Ingredients

- 0.5 scoops Stevia
- 0.5 cups oats
- A pinch of Cloves
- 1 Tbsp Walnuts
- A pinch of Nutmeg
- 0.25 tsp Vanilla extract
- 1 tsp Molasses
- 2 tsp Chia seeds
- A pinch of Ginger
- A pinch of Cinnamon
- 0.5 cups vanilla almond milk

Procedure

1. Combine all ingredients, except the walnuts, in a sealed container until thoroughly mixed.
2. Refrigerate overnight.
3. Top with walnuts and serve.

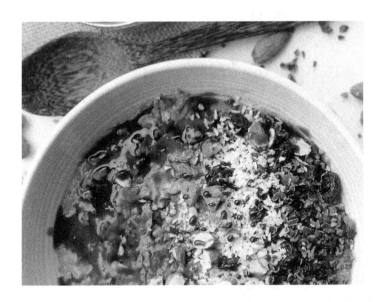

Peach Smoothie

Serves 1 pax

Ingredients

- 0.5 cups Crushed ice
- 1 tsp sweetener
- 1 Peach
- 1 Tbsp Orange juice concentrate
- 0.5 cups Milk

Procedure

1. Toss each of the fixings into a blender.
2. Mix until it's all creamy smooth.
3. Serve it promptly.

Breakfast Burritos

Serves 4 pax

Ingredients

- 4 tsp Salsa
- 4 Corn tortillas
- 8 Eggs
- 1 Avocado
- 0.25 cups Bell pepper
- 1 tsp Black pepper
- 2 Tbsp cheddar cheese
- 0.25 cups Onion
- 3 ounces Reduced-sodium ham
- 2 tsp Margarine
- 1 tbsp Hot sauce

Procedure

1. Gather a large mixing container and whisk four whole eggs and four egg whites (reserving the yolks for another time) with the pepper, hot sauce, and cheese.
2. Prepare a non-stick skillet using the medium temperature setting to melt the margarine.
3. Cook the ham for 2 to 3 minutes. Place the ham aside.
4. Put the onion and bell pepper in the hot pan. Cook them using the medium temperature setting for approximately 5 minutes.
5. Mix in the cooked ham and decrease the heat to low.
6. Empty the egg mixture into the pan and cook, continuously stirring, until the eggs are fully cooked.
7. Remove pan from heat.
8. Serve warm.

Gluten-Free ChocoBanana Muffins

Serves 14 pax

Ingredients

- 0.5 cups Cocoa powder
- 2 Very ripe bananas
- 0.5 cups Sugar
- 0.25 cups Water
- 2 Tbsp Mini chocolate chips
- 1 Tbsp Water
- 2 Eggs
- 1 tsp Vanilla extract
- 0.5 cups Quinoa flakes
- 1 cup Gluten-free baking mix - all-purpose

Procedure

1. Set the oven at 350° Fahrenheit.
2. Whisk the oil, sugar, and vanilla in a large bowl. One at a time, mix in the bananas and eggs, mixing after each addition. Mix in the baking mix, quinoa flakes, cocoa powder, and water.
3. Spoon the batter into 14 muffin cups lined with muffin papers and sprayed with nonstick spray. Divide the chocolate chips evenly on top of each muffin.
4. Bake until a toothpick inserted in the center comes out clean (20-22 min.).
5. Be sure to cool the muffins in the pan for about ten minutes, then place on a wire rack to thoroughly cool, but they can also be eaten warm.

Green Manchego Salad

Serves 6 pax

Ingredients

- 1 teaspoon Dijon mustard
- 4 ounces Manchego cheese
- 6 cups mesclun greens
- Salt and pepper to taste to taste
- 1/4 cup extra-virgin olive oil
- 1/3 cup almonds
- 1 shallot
- 5 teaspoons sherry vinegar

Procedure

1. Place mesclun in a big container. Beat vinegar, shallot, mustard, 1/4 teaspoon salt, and 1/4 teaspoon pepper together in a small-sized container. Whisking continuously, slowly drizzle in oil.
2. Sprinkle vinaigrette over mesclun and gently toss to coat.
3. Sprinkle with Salt and pepper to taste to taste.
4. Serve, topping individual portions with almonds and Manchego.

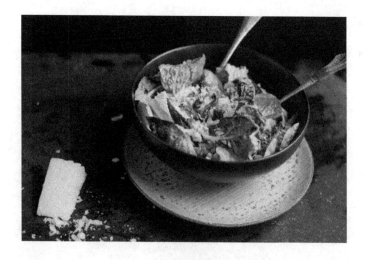

Breakfast Egg Cups

Serves 6 pax

Ingredients

- 1 cup Egg substitute
- 2 Tbsp Monterey Jack cheese
- 2 Tbsp Turkey bacon Black pepper
- 0.25 tsp Salt
- 1 clove Garlic
- 3 turkey sausage patties
- 2 Tbsp Light sour cream tsp Canola oil
- 1.25 cups Hash browns
- 2 Tbsp Onion

Procedure

1. Spray a 6-cavity muffin pan with nonstick spray. Evenly divide the hash browns between the cups and press them on the base and up the sides of each cup.

2. Warm the oil in a large frying pan using the medium temperature setting. Sauté the onion until translucent.

3. Stir in the garlic and sausage and cook for one more minute. Transfer the skillet to a cool burner and mix in the sour cream.

4. Mix the Salt and pepper to taste into the egg substitute.

5. Pour it evenly into the muffin cups, then top with the sausage mixture, bacon, and cheese.

6. Bake at 400°F until the eggs are no longer jiggly and wet, about 15 to 18 minutes.

7. Serve it.

Pancake Puffs

Serves 2 pax

Ingredients

- 1 tsp Salt
- 2 Tbsp All-purpose flour
- 0.25 cups egg
- 2 Tbsp Mixed berry yogurt
- 6 Strawberries
- oz Raspberries
- 0.25 tsp Vanilla extract
- 2 tsp Canola oil
- 2 Tbsp Skim milk

Procedure

1. Mix the egg substitute, flour, milk, oil, vanilla extract, and salt until smooth.
2. Divide the batter between two 4" ramekins coated in cooking spray.
3. Bake the ramekins on a baking sheet at 400°F until golden brown and puffy (2025 min.).
4. Transfer the pan to the countertop and pierce each puff with the tip of a knife. Let rest for 5 minutes while you mix the strawberries and raspberries.
5. Place half of the berries on each puff, then top each with 1 Tbsp. yogurt.
6. Serve.

Berries with Cream

Serves 4 pax

Ingredients

- 2 cups Strawberries
- 0.5 cups vanilla pudding
- 2 cups Blueberries
- 4 Tbsp Light whipped topping

Procedure

1. Stir together the pudding and whipped topping in a small-sized mixing container.
2. Use another container to combine the blueberries and strawberries.
3. Place 1 cup of berries in each of 4 small dessert dishes and top each with 2.5 Tbsp. pudding mixture.

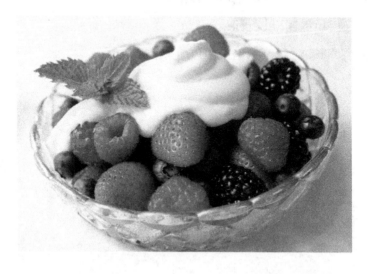

Overnight Peanut Butter Oats

Serves 2 pax

Ingredients

- 2 oz Whole milk
- 1 cup Strawberries or peaches
- 2 tsp Vanilla extract
- 2 Tbsp Peanut butter
- Half Banana
- Half oz Whole oats
- 3 Tbsp Chia seeds

Procedure

1. In a resealable dish, pour in milk, chia seeds, peanut butter, and banana. Stir to combine.
2. Include the oats and stir them to coat evenly with the peanut butter mixture.
3. Seal and place in the fridge overnight.
4. When sitting down to eat, top with fruit and serve.

Almond Flour Cookies

Serves 10 pax

Ingredients

- 4 oz Butter
- 3 oz Powdered erythritol
- 2 tsp Almond extract
- 4 oz Almond flour
- 5 Eggs

Procedure

1. Cookies bake best at 350° F, so prepare your oven accordingly.
2. Whip the erythritol powder and butter. Crack in the eggs, mixing until smooth.
3. Stir in the almond extract and almond flour slowly.
4. Once fully incorporated, roll the dough into 20 cookies.
5. Place parchment paper on a baking sheet and arrange your cookies without the edges touching.
6. Bake for 15 minutes. Once the edges of the cookies are crispy, remove from the oven.
7. Allow the cookies time for cooling before serving.

Avocado Crab Boats

Serves 8 pax

Ingredients

- 3 Tbsp Chives
- 2 Tbsp Fresh cilantro
- 5 Avocados
- 2 Tbsp Capers
- 2 Tbsp Lemon juice
- 4 Lemon wedges
- 12 oz Lump crabmeat
- A quarter tsp black pepper
- 1 tsp Pepper jack cheese
- 2 tbsp Mayonnaise
- half tsp Paprika
- 1 Serrano pepper

Procedure

1. Set your oven to broil. Place two avocado halves in a bowl and mash them.
2. Scoop in the mayonnaise and pour in the lemon juice. Mix well.
3. Stir in the crab, three tablespoons of the cilantro, serrano pepper, chives, capers, and black pepper.
4. Spoon the mixture into the remaining eight avocado halves.
5. Move the boats onto a baking sheet that has been covered with parchment.
6. Sprinkle paprika, then shredded cheese onto each avocado boat.
7. Place the sheet into the oven and broil for four minutes, waiting for the cheese to become bubbly and melted.
8. Remove from heat and top with the remaining cilantro.
9. Serve with lemon wedges and serve.

Ham and Springtime Salad

Serves 6 pax

Ingredients

- 2 teaspoons raspberry vinegar
- 3 tablespoons olive oil
- 2 tablespoons orange juice
- 1 teaspoon coarse grained prepared mustard
- 1/2 cup diced peaches, drained
- 1 red onion, thinly sliced
- Ground black pepper to taste
- 3 cups cooked ham, cubed
- 8 cups baby spinach, rinsed and dried
- 1 cup diced cantaloupe

Procedure

1. Whisk together pepper, mustard, vinegar, juice and oil in a small bowl.

2. Toss together onion, peaches, cantaloupe, spinach and ham in a large bowl.

3. Drizzle dressing over salad and toss until well coated.

4. Serve right away.

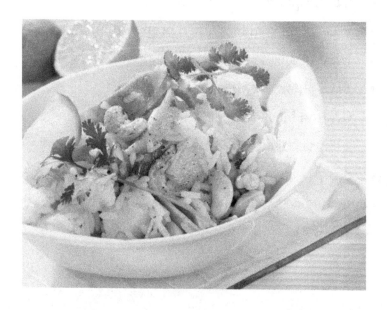

Guacamole

Serves 2 pax

Ingredients

- 2 tbsp Chunky salsa
- 1 tsp Salt
- 2 Avocados
- 1 Tbsp Lemon juice

Procedure

1. Take the avocados, remove the skin, and chop into cubes. Place the cubes into a bowl.
2. Squeeze the lemon juice and stir in the salsa and salt. Mash with a fork.
3. Put nicely on a serving dish and serve.

Homemade Granola

Serves 4 pax

Ingredients

- 0.25 oz Coconut oil
- 0.25 oz Maple syrup
- 1 oz Raisins
- 2 oz Whole oats
- Half oz Almonds
- 0.5 tsp Vanilla extract
- 0.25 tsp Cinnamon

Procedure

1. Set your oven to 350° F and shield your baking sheet with parchment paper.

2. Taking a large container, incorporate your nuts and oats. Toss with cinnamon and salt. Stir well.

3. Combine in the oil, vanilla, and syrup while stirring. Combine well, coating everything.

4. Dump your granola onto your baking sheet and spread it into a flat layer with a large spoon. If the layer is piled up too much, move it to a second sheet.

5. Put it into the oven for 20 minutes, stirring halfway through.

6. Pull granola out of the oven and wait for it to cool for 45 minutes to harden. When cooled, toss your raisins on top.

7. Break apart the granola with your hands into chunks the size that you want.

Melba Toast

Serves 4 pax

Ingredients

- 1/8 teaspoon dried dill
- 1 tablespoon unsalted butter, melted
- 4 slices of fresh baked white bread
- 1/8 teaspoon dried thyme

Procedure

1. Preheat oven to 350°F. Mix melted butter, dill and thyme in a small bowl. Add Salt and pepper to taste to taste.

2. Roll bread very thin with a rolling pin. Trim off crusts. Brush bread with the butter mixture both sides

3. Cut slice diagonally into triangles. Place the triangles on a baking sheet on the center rack of oven.

4. Bake 15 minutes, turning halfway through. Toasts are done when browned and crisp.

5. Cool the toasts on a rack and serve with salad.

Berry Parfaits

Serves 6 pax

Ingredients

- Half oz Raspberries
- 2 oz Granola
- 32 oz Vanilla Greek yogurt
- 2 oz Strawberries
- 2 oz Blueberries

Procedure

1. Take your berries and mix them all together. Set up 6 bowls, mason jars, or Tupperware with lids.
2. Spoon in your mixed berries, followed by a layer of yogurt.
3. Continue to alternate evenly until all ingredients are used. Then, portion granola into 1/4 c. servings in their own zipper seal bags to top when ready to eat.
4. Serve by stirring the granola mixture into the yogurt parfait.

Spinach and Mint Salad

Serves 2 pax

Ingredients

- 1 cup sliced avocado
- 1/2 cup diced red bell pepper
- 4 cups fresh spinach leaves
- 3 tablespoons vegetable oil
- 1 clove garlic, minced
- 1 cup sliced cantaloupe
- 2 tablespoons chopped fresh mint leaves
- 1 tablespoon mint apple jelly
- 1 teaspoon white wine vinegar

Procedure

4. Distribute spinach to 2 serving plates. Put half of each avocado and half of the cantaloupe on spinach in a circle pattern on every plate.
5. Top with fresh mint and diced red pepper.
6. Mix garlic, oil, white wine vinegar and mint jelly. Drizzle on salads.
7. Serve.

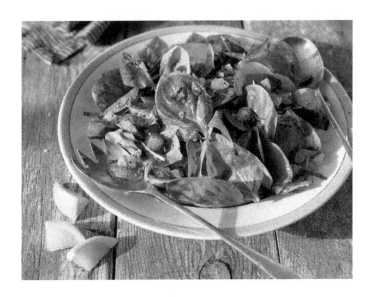

Blue Cheese Potato Salad

Serves 5 pax

Ingredients

- 1/2 cup olive oil
- 3 tablespoons white vinegar
- 5 slices bacon
- 1 teaspoon ground black pepper
- 2 ounces blue cheese, crumbled
- 2 pounds red new potatoes
- 1 bunch green onions, chopped
- 1/2 teaspoon salt

Procedure

1. In a large, deep skillet, fry bacon over medium-high heat until browned evenly.

2. Remove from fat, chop into small pieces and set aside.

3. Salt the water in a large pot then bring water to a boil. Pour potatoes and cook for about 15 minutes until tender, but still firm.

4. Drain off water, allow to cool and chop, do not remove the skins.

5. Combine pepper, salt, green onions, vinegar, and oil together in a large bowl.

6. Add cheese, bacon, and potatoes then gently shake to coat.

7. Serve.

Oatmeal Cookies

Serves 6 pax

Ingredients

- 0.5 tsp Baking soda
- 1 Banana
- Half oz Almond butter
- Half oz Almond flour
- 0.25 oz Walnuts
- 1 oz Whole oats
- 0.5 tsp Baking powder
- Half oz Blueberries
- 0.5 tsp Cinnamon
- 0.25 oz Coconut oil
- 1 Egg
- 1 Lemon
- 2 oz Oat flour
- 0.5 tsp Salt
- 1 tsp Vanilla extract

Procedure

1. Your oven should be prepared to 350F. Then, cover a sheet pan with parchment.
2. Using a small container, whisk an egg until it begins to froth.
3. In a separate one, combine your flours, oats, baking soda and powder, salt, lemon zest, and cinnamon. Mix well until fully incorporated.
4. In a third container, combine your oil, butter, and banana, combining well.
5. Mix your egg into your almond butter mixture.
6. Then, take the almond butter mixture and slowly combine it into your flour mixture until you get a thick cookie batter.
7. When mixed well, gently combine in your blueberries and walnuts.
8. Put the batter into 12 evenly sized cookies.
9. Bake until the edges start to brown, roughly 20 minutes. The centers should be soft. Take them out and allow them to cool for 5 minutes.
10. Serve.

Boiled Eggs

Serves 6 pax

Ingredients

- 6 Eggs
- A pinch of Salt
- 1 cup Vinegar Water

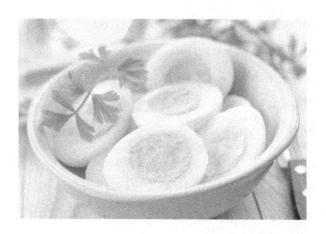

Procedure

1. Begin by placing eggs into a big pot. Then, cover the eggs up with water entirely.
2. Sprinkle salt and splash in a bit of vinegar into the water to make them easier to peel later on.
3. Turn on and bring the eggs to a boil. From there, how long you keep them in the boiling water is dependent upon how to set you want your yolks to be.
4. 3 minutes for soft-boiled eggs—perfect for use in a savory ramen.
5. 6 minutes for medium-boiled eggs—perfect for enjoying as is.
6. Twelve minutes for hard-boiled eggs—perfect for a sandwich or something similar.
7. When your eggs have boiled long enough, you need to bring them to a cool as quickly as possible, so they don't overcook. To do so, transfer your eggs to an ice bath.
8. To peel them, crack gently on a table, then peel.
9. These can be kept in the fridge for easy snacks on the go, or you can eat them right away.

Brown Feta

Serves 10 pax

Ingredients

- 8 ounces feta cheese
- 1/4 teaspoon red pepper flakes
- 3 tablespoons extra-virgin olive oil
- 2 teaspoons parsley
- 1/4 teaspoon pepper

Procedure

1. Place oven rack 4 inches from broiler element and heat broiler.
2. Pat feta dry using paper towels and lay out on broiler-safe gratin dish.
3. Drizzle with red pepper flakes and pepper.
4. Broil until edges of cheese start to look golden, three to eight minutes.
5. Sprinkle with oil, drizzle with parsley, and serve instantly.

Spinach and Mushroom Omelet

Serves 2 pax

Ingredients

- 1 Onion
- 2 Tbsp Olive oil
- 3 Mushrooms
- 0.25 tsp Black pepper
- 1 Egg
- 1 oz Spinach
- 1 Tbsp Milk
- 0.5 tsp Garlic powder

Procedure

1. Warm a big pan over medium heat and toss in the oil. Then, heat your mushroom and onion for 3 minutes until tender, giving it an occasional stir. Warm for 1 minute until spinach wilts. Then, remove the veggies and place them aside.

2. Take a medium bowl and combine your egg substitute, milk, garlic powder, and pepper. Combine well.

3. Then, coat your pan with cooking spray and return it to medium heat. Toss in your egg mixture and stir gently for a minute, then allow it to set.

4. Top the eggs with the veggie mixture and carefully fold the omelet in half, sliding it onto your platter.

5. Serve immediately.

Thanks

To all of you who arrived until here.

I am glad you accepted my teachings.
These have been my personal meals in the past years, so I wished to share them with you.

Now you had come to know about Salads and Healthy brunches, let me give you one more tip.
This manual takes part of an unmissable cookbooks collection.
These salad-based recipes, mixed to all the tastes I met in my worldwide journeys, will give you a complete idea of the possibilities this world offers to us.
You have now the opportunity to add hundreds new elements to your cooking skills knowledge.
Check out the other books!

CPSIA information can be obtained
at www.ICGtesting.com
Printed in the USA
BVHW041101130521
607269BV00012B/2514